The Definitive Keto Cookbool

Get Ready to Prepare the Quick and Eas
Diet

Skye Webb

Table of contents

Black Bean Taco Salad Bowl

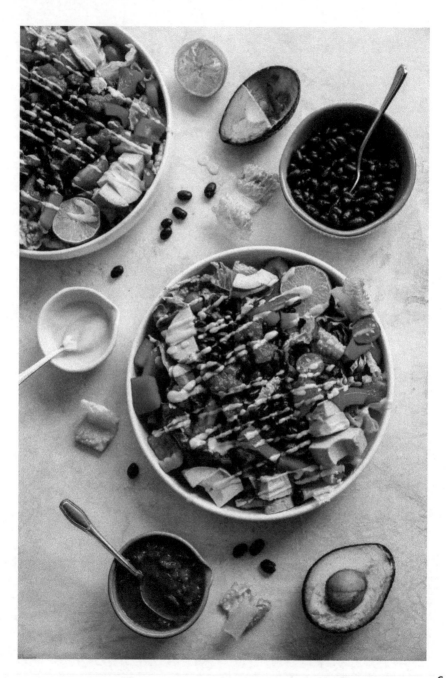

Preparation time: 15 minutes cooking time: 5 minutes servings: 3

Ingredients

For the black bean salad

1 (14-ouncecan black beans, drained and rinsed, or 1½ cups cooked 1 cup corn kernels, fresh and blanched, or frozen and thawed

¼ cup fresh cilantro, or parsley, chopped Zest and juice of 1 lime

1 to 2 teaspoons chili powder Pinch sea salt

1½ cups cherry tomatoes, halved

1 red bell pepper, seeded and chopped 2 scallions, chopped

For 1 serving of tortilla chips

1 large whole-grain tortilla or wrap

1 teaspoon olive oil

Pinch sea salt

Pinch freshly ground black pepper Pinch dried oregano

Pinch chili powder For 1 bowl

1 cup fresh greens (lettuce, spinach, or whatever you like

¾ cup cooked quinoa, or brown rice, millet, or other whole grain

¼ cup chopped avocado, or Guacamole

¼ cup Fresh Mango Salsa

Directions

To Make The Black Bean Salad

1.   Toss All The Ingredients Together In A Large Bowl.

2.   To Make The Tortilla Chips

3.   Brush The Tortilla With Olive Oil, Then Sprinkle With Salt, Pepper, Oregano, Chili Powder, And Any Other Seasonings You Like. Slice It Into Eighths Like A Pizza.

4.   Transfer The Tortilla Pieces To A Small Baking Sheet Lined With Parchment Paper And Put In The Oven Or Toaster Oven To Toast Or Broil For 3 To 5 Minutes, Until Browned. Keep An Eye On Them, As They Can Go From Just Barely Done To Burned Very Quickly.

To Make The Bowl

5.   Lay The Greens In The Bowl, Top With The Cooked Quinoa, ⅓ Of The Black Bean Salad, The Avocado, And Salsa.

Nutrition: Calories: 589; Total fat: 14g; Carbs: 101g; Fiber: 20g; Protein: 21g

4

Romaine And Grape Tomato Salad With Avocado And Baby Peas

Preparation time: 15 minutes cooking time: 0 minutes servings: 4

Ingredients

1 garlic clove, chopped

1 tablespoon chopped shallot ½ teaspoon dried basil

½ teaspoon salt

⅛ teaspoon freshly ground black pepper ¼ teaspoon brown sugar (optional

3 tablespoons white wine vinegar ⅓ cup olive oil

1 medium head romaine lettuce, cut into ¼-inch strips 12 ripe grape tomatoes, halved

½ cup frozen baby peas, thawed 8 kalamata olives, pitted

1 ripe Hass avocado

Directions

1.   In a blender or food processor, combine the garlic, shallot, basil, salt, pepper, sugar, and vinegar until smooth. Add the oil and blend until emulsified. Set aside.

2.   In a large bowl, combine the lettuce, tomatoes, peas, and olives. Pit and peel the avocado and cut into ½-inch dice. Add to the bowl, along with enough dressing to lightly coat. Toss gently to combine and serve.

Warm Vegetable "Salad"

Preparation time: 10 minutes cooking time: 15 minutes

servings: 4

Ingredients

Salt for salting water, plus ½ teaspoon (optional 4 red potatoes, quartered

1   pound carrots, sliced into ¼-inch-thick rounds

1 tablespoon extra-virgin olive oil (optional

2   tablespoons lime juice

2 teaspoons dried dill

¼ teaspoon freshly ground black pepper

1   cup Cashew Cream or Parm-y Kale Pesto

Directions

1.   In a large pot, bring salted water to a boil. Add the potatoes and cook for 8 minutes. Add the carrots and continue to boil for another 8 minutes, until both the potatoes and carrots are crisp tender. Drain and return to the pot. Add the olive oil (if using), lime juice, dill, remaining ½ teaspoon of salt (if using), and pepper, and stir to coat well.

2.   Divide the vegetables evenly among 4 single-compartment storage containers or wide-mouth pint glass jars, and spoon ¼

cup of cream or pesto over the vegetables in each. Let cool before sealing the lids.

Nutrition: Calories: 393; Fat: 15g; Protein: 10g; Carbohydrates: 52g; Fiber: 9g; Sugar: 8g; Sodium: 343mg

Puttanesca Seitan And Spinach Salad

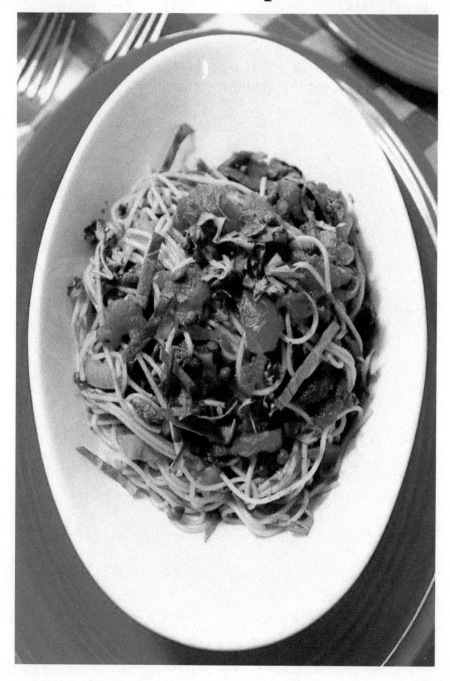

Preparation time: 5 minutes cooking time: 6 minutes servings: 4

Ingredients

4 tablespoons olive oil

8 ounces seitan, homemade or store-bought, cut into ½-inch strips

3 garlic cloves, minced

½ cup kalamata olives, pitted and halved

½ cup green olives, pitted and halved

2   tablespoons capers

3   cups fresh baby spinach, cut into strips

1½ cups ripe cherry tomatoes, halved

2 tablespoons balsamic vinegar

¼ teaspoon salt (optional

¼ teaspoon freshly ground black pepper

2 tablespoons torn fresh basil leaves

2   tablespoons minced fresh parsley

Directions

1.   In a large skillet, heat 1 tablespoon of the oil over medium heat. Add the seitan and cook until browned on both sides, about 5 minutes. Add the garlic and cook until fragrant, about 30 seconds. Transfer to a large bowl and set aside to cool, about 15 minutes.

2.   When the seitan has cooled to room temperature, add the kalamata and green olives, capers, spinach, and tomatoes. Set aside.

3.   In a small bowl, combine the remaining 3 tablespoons oil with the vinegar, salt, and pepper. Whisk until blended, then pour the dressing over the salad. Add the basil and parsley, toss gently to combine, and serve.

Rice Salad With Cashews And Dried Papaya

Preparation time: 15 minutes cooking time: 0 minutes servings: 4

Ingredients

3½ cups cooked brown rice

½ cup chopped roasted cashews ½ cup thinly sliced dried papaya 4 green onions, chopped

3   tablespoons fresh lime juice 2 teaspoons agave nectar

1 teaspoon grated fresh ginger ⅓ cup grapeseed oil

Salt and freshly ground black pepper

Directions

1.   In a large bowl, combine the rice, cashews, papaya, and green onions. Set aside.

2.   In a small bowl, combine the lime juice, agave nectar, and ginger. Whisk in the oil and season with the salt and pepper to taste. Pour the dressing over the rice mixture, mix well, and serve.

Spinach Salad With Orange-Dijon Dressing

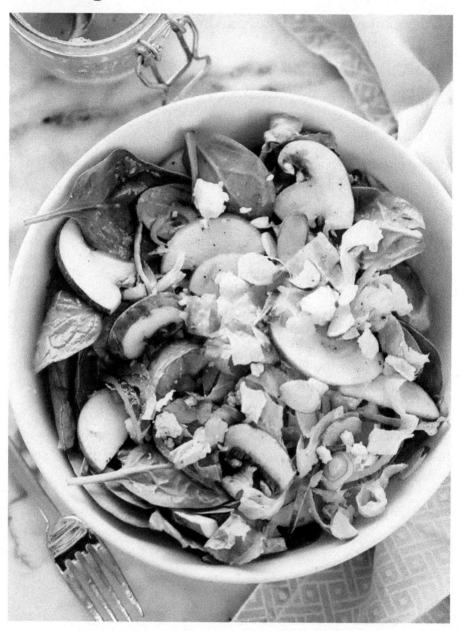

Preparation time: 10 minutes cooking time: 0 minutes servings: 4

Ingredients

2 tablespoons Dijon mustard

2 tablespoons olive oil

1⁄4 cup fresh orange juice

1 teaspoon agave nectar

1⁄2 teaspoon salt

1⁄4 teaspoon freshly ground black pepper

2 tablespoons minced fresh parsley

1 tablespoon minced green onions

5 cups fresh baby spinach, torn into bite-size pieces

1 navel orange, peeled and segmented

1⁄2 small red onion, sliced paper thin

Directions

1.   In a blender or food processor combine the mustard, oil, orange juice, agave nectar, salt, pepper, parsley, and green onions. Blend well and set aside.

2.   In a large bowl, combine the spinach, orange, and onion. Add the dressing, toss gently to combine, and serve.

Caramelized Onion And Beet Salad

Preparation time: 10 minutes cooking time: 40 minutes servings: 4

Ingredients

3 medium golden beets

2 cups sliced sweet or Vidalia onions

1   teaspoon extra-virgin olive oil or no-beef broth

Pinch baking soda

¼ to ½ teaspoon salt, to taste

2   tablespoons unseasoned rice vinegar, white wine vinegar, or balsamic vinegar

Directions

1.   Cut the greens off the beets, and scrub the beets.

2.   In a large pot, place a steamer basket and fill the pot with 2 inches of water.

3.   Add the beets, bring to a boil, then reduce the heat to medium, cover, and steam for about 35 minutes, until you can easily pierce the middle of the beets with a knife.

4.   Meanwhile, in a large, dry skillet over medium heat, sauté the onions for 5 minutes, stirring frequently.

5.   Add the olive oil and baking soda, and continuing cooking for 5 more minutes, stirring frequently. Stir in the salt to taste before removing from the heat. Transfer to a large bowl and set aside.

6.   When the beets have cooked through, drain and cool until easy to handle. Rub the beets in a paper towel to easily remove the skins. Cut into wedges, and transfer to the bowl with the onions. Drizzle the vinegar over everything and toss well.

7.   Divide the beets evenly among 4 wide-mouth jars or storage containers. Let cool before sealing the lids.

Nutrition: Calories: 104; Fat: 2g; Protein: 3g; Carbohydrates: 20g; Fiber: 4g; Sugar: 14g; Sodium: 303mg

Treasure Barley Salad

Preparation time: 10 minutes cooking time: 30 minutes servings: 4 to 6

Ingredients

1 cup pearl barley

1½ cups cooked or 1 (15.5-ouncecan navy beans, drained and rinsed 1 celery rib, finely chopped

1 medium carrot, shredded 3 green onions, minced

½ cup chopped pitted kalamata olives

½ cup dried cherries or sweetened dried cranberries ½ cup toasted pecans pieces, coarsely chopped

½ cup minced fresh parsley 1 garlic clove, pressed

3   tablespoons sherry vinegar

Salt and freshly ground black pepper

¼ cup grapeseed oil

Directions

1.   In a large saucepan, bring 2½ cups salted water to boil over high heat. Add the barley and return to a boil. Reduce heat to low, cover, and simmer until the barley is tender, about 30 minutes. Transfer to a serving bowl.

2.   Add the beans, celery, carrot, green onions, olives, cherries, pecans, and parsley. Set aside.

3.　　In a small bowl, combine the garlic, vinegar, and salt and pepper to taste. Whisk in the oil until well blended. Pour the dressing over the salad, toss to combine, and serve.

Golden Couscous Salad

Preparation time: 5 minutes cooking time: 12 minutes servings: 4

Ingredients

1/4 cup olive oil

1   medium shallot, minced

1/2 teaspoon ground coriander

1/2 teaspoon turmeric

1/4 teaspoon ground cayenne

1 cup couscous

2   cups vegetable broth, homemade or store-bought, or water
Salt

1   medium yellow bell pepper, chopped

1 medium carrot, shredded

1/2 cup chopped dried apricots 1/4 cup golden raisins

1/4 cup chopped unsalted roasted cashews

11/2 cups cooked or 1 (15.5-ouncecan chickpeas, drained and rinsed 2 tablespoons minced fresh cilantro leaves

2   tablespoons fresh lemon juice

 Directions

1.   In a large saucepan, heat 1 tablespoon of the oil over medium heat. Add the shallot, coriander, turmeric, cayenne, and couscous and stir until fragrant, about 2 minutes, being careful not to burn. Stir in the broth and salt to taste. Bring to a boil, then remove from the heat, cover, and let stand for 10 minutes.

2.   Transfer the cooked couscous to a large bowl. Add the bell pepper, carrot, apricots, raisins, cashews, chickpeas, and cilantro. Toss gently to combine and set aside.

3.   In a small bowl, combine the remaining 3 tablespoons of oil with the lemon juice, stirring to blend. Pour the dressing over the salad, toss gently to combine, and serve.

Chopped Salad

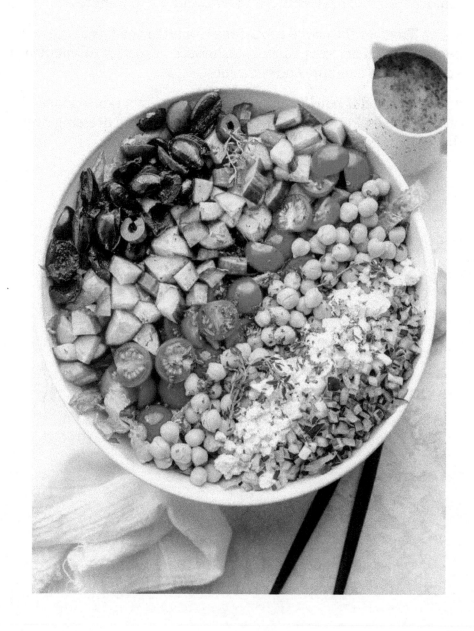

Preparation time: 15 minutes cooking time: 0 minutes servings: 4

Ingredients

¾ cup olive oil

¼ cup white wine vinegar 2 teaspoons

Dijon mustard 1 garlic clove

1 tablespoon minced green onions

 ½ teaspoon salt (optional

¼ teaspoon ground black pepper

½ small head romaine lettuce, chopped ½ small head iceberg lettuce, chopped

1½ cups cooked or 1 (15.5-ouncecan chickpeas, drained and rinsed 2 ripe tomatoes, cut into ½-inch dice

1 medium English cucumber, peeled, halved lengthwise, and chopped 2 celery ribs, chopped celery

1   medium carrot, chopped

½ cup halved pitted kalamata olives 3 small red radishes, chopped

2   tablespoons chopped fresh parsley

1 ripe Hass avocado, pitted, peeled, and cut into ½-inch dice

Directions

1.   In a blender or food processor, combine the oil, vinegar, mustard, garlic, green onions, salt, and pepper. Blend well and set aside.

2.   In a large bowl, combine the romaine and iceberg lettuces. Add the chickpeas, tomatoes, cucumber, celery, carrot, olives, radishes, parsley, and avocado. Add enough dressing to lightly coat. Toss gently to combine and serve.

Warm Lentil Salad with Red Wine Vinaigrette

Preparation time: 10 minutes cooking time: 50 minutes servings: 4

Ingredients

1 teaspoon olive oil plus ¼ cup, divided, or 1 tablespoon vegetable broth or water 1 small onion, diced

1 garlic clove, minced

1 carrot, diced

1 cup lentils

1 tablespoon dried basil

1 tablespoon dried oregano

1   tablespoon red wine or balsamic vinegar (optional 2 cups water

¼ cup red wine vinegar or balsamic vinegar

1 teaspoon sea salt

2   cups chopped Swiss chard

2 cups torn red leaf lettuce

4 tablespoons Cheesy Sprinkle

Directions

1.   Heat 1 teaspoon of the oil in a large pot on medium heat, then sauté the onion and garlic until they are translucent, about 5 minutes.

2.　　Add the carrot and sauté until it is slightly cooked, about 3 minutes. Stir in the lentils, basil, and oregano, then add the wine or balsamic vinegar (if using).

3.　　Pour the water into the pot and turn the heat up to high to bring to a boil.

4.　　Turn the heat down to a simmer and let the lentils cook, uncovered, 20 to 30 minutes, until they are soft but not falling apart.

5.　　While the lentils are cooking, whisk together the red wine vinegar, olive oil, and salt in a small bowl and set aside. Once the lentils have cooked, drain any excess liquid and stir in most of the red wine vinegar dressing. Set a little bit of dressing aside. Add the Swiss chard to the pot and stir it into the lentils. Leave the heat on low and cook, stirring, for at least 10 minutes. Toss the lettuce with the

remaining dressing. Place some lettuce on a plate, and top with the lentil mixture. Finish the plate off with a little Cheesy Sprinkle and enjoy.

Nutrition Calories: 387; Total fat: 17g; Carbs: 42g; Fiber: 19g; Protein: 18g

Carrot And Orange Salad With Cashews And Cilantro

Preparation time: 15 minutes cooking time: 0 minutes servings: 4

Ingredients

1   pound carrots, shredded

2   oranges, peeled, segmented, and chopped ½ cup unsalted roasted cashews

¼ cup chopped fresh cilantro

2 tablespoons fresh orange juice 2 tablespoons fresh lime juice

2 teaspoons brown sugar (optional

Salt (optional) and freshly ground black pepper ⅓ cup olive oil

Directions

1.   In a large bowl, combine the carrots, oranges, cashews, and cilantro and set aside.

2.   In a small bowl, combine the orange juice, lime juice, sugar, and salt and pepper to taste. Whisk in the oil until blended. Pour the dressing over the carrot mixture, stirring to lightly coat. Taste, adjusting seasonings if necessary. Toss gently to combine and serve.

Not-Tuna Salad

Preparation time: 5 minutes cooking time: 0 minutes servings: 4

Ingredients

1 (15.5-ouncecan chickpeas, drained and rinsed

1 (14-ouncecan hearts of palm, drained and chopped

½ cup chopped yellow or white onion

½ cup diced celery

¼ cup vegan mayonnaise, plus more if needed

½ teaspoon salt

¼ teaspoon freshly ground black pepper

Directions

1. In a medium bowl, use a potato masher or fork to roughly mash the chickpeas until chunky and "shredded." Add the hearts of palm, onion, celery, vegan mayonnaise, salt, and pepper.

2. Combine and add more mayonnaise, if necessary, for a creamy texture. Into each of 4 single-serving containers, place ¾ cup of salad. Seal the lids.

Nutrition: Calories: 214; Fat: 6g; Protein: 9g; Carbohydrates: 35g; Fiber: 8g; Sugar: 1g; Sodium: 765mg

Dazzling Vegetable Salad

Preparation time: 15 minutes cooking time: 0 minutes

servings: 4

Ingredients

1 medium carrot, shredded

1 cup finely shredded red cabbage

1 cup ripe grape or cherry tomatoes, halved

1 medium yellow bell pepper, cut into matchsticks

1½ cups cooked or 1 (15.5-ouncecan chickpeas, rinsed and drained ¼ cup halved pitted kalamata olives

1   ripe Hass avocado, pitted, peeled, and cut into ½-inch dice ¼ cup olive oil

1½ tablespoons fresh lemon juice ½ teaspoon salt

⅛ teaspoon freshly ground black pepper Pinch sugar (optional

Directions

1.   In a large bowl, combine the watercress, carrot, cabbage, tomatoes, bell pepper, chickpeas, olives, and avocado and set

aside.

2.   In a small bowl, combine the oil, lemon juice, salt, black pepper, and sugar. Blend well and add to the salad. Toss gently to combine and serve.

Red Bean and Corn Salad

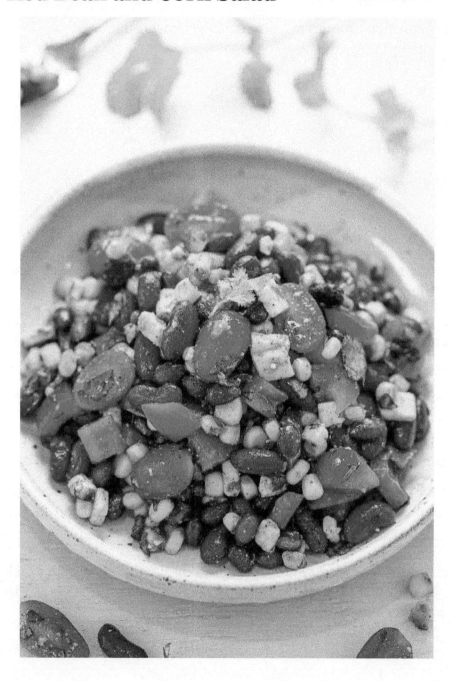

Preparation time: 15 minutes cooking time: 0 minutes servings: 4

Ingredients

¼ cup Cashew Cream or other salad dressing

1 teaspoon chili powder

2   (14.5-ouncecans kidney beans, rinsed and drained

2 cups frozen corn, thawed, or 2 cups canned corn, drained

1 cup cooked farro, barley, or rice (optional

8 cups chopped romaine lettuce

Directions

1.   Line up 4 wide-mouth glass quart jars.

2.   In a small bowl, whisk the cream and chili powder. Pour 1 tablespoon of cream into each jar. In each jar, add ¾ cup kidney beans, ½ cup corn, ¼ cup cooked farro (if using), and 2 cups romaine, punching it down to fit it into the jar. Close the lids tightly.

Nutrition: Calories: 303; Fat: 9g; Protein: 14g; Carbohydrates: 45g; Fiber: 15g; Sugar: 6g; Sodium: 654mg

Mango And Snow Pea Salad

Preparation time: 15 minutes cooking time: 0 minutes servings: 4

Ingredients

½ teaspoon minced garlic

½ teaspoon grated fresh ginger

¼ cup creamy peanut butter

1 tablespoon plus 1 teaspoon light brown sugar

¼ teaspoon crushed red pepper

3 tablespoons rice vinegar 3 tablespoons water

1   tablespoon soy sauce

2   cups snow peas, trimmed and lightly blanched

2 ripe mangos, peeled, pitted, cut into ½-inch dice 1 large carrot, shredded

1   medium cucumber, peeled, halved lengthwise, and seeded 3 cups shredded romaine lettuce

½ cup chopped unsalted roasted peanuts, for garnish

Directions

1.   In a small bowl, combine the garlic, ginger, peanut butter, sugar, and crushed red pepper. Stir in the vinegar, water, and soy sauce. Taste, adjusting seasonings, if necessary, and set aside.

2.   Cut the snow peas diagonally into a thin matchsticks and place in a large bowl. Add the mangos and carrot. Cut the cucumber into ¼-inch slices and add to the bowl.

3.   Pour the dressing onto the salad and toss gently to combine. Spoon the salad onto a bed of shredded lettuce, sprinkle with peanuts, and serve.

Cucumber-Radish Salad With Tarragon Vinaigrette

Preparation time: 15 minutes cooking time: 0 minutes servings: 4

Ingredients

2   medium English cucumbers, peeled, halved, seeded, cut into 1/4-inch slices 6 small red radishes, cut into 1/8-inch slices

2 1/2 tablespoons tarragon vinegar 1/2 teaspoon dried tarragon

1/4 teaspoon sugar

Salt and freshly ground black pepper 1/4 cup olive oil

Directions

1.   In a large bowl, combine the cucumbers and the radishes and set aside.

2.   In a small bowl, combine the vinegar, tarragon, sugar, and salt and pepper to taste. Whisk in the oil until well blended, then add the dressing to the salad. Toss gently to combine and serve.

Italian-Style Pasta Salad

Preparation time: 5 minutes cooking time: 10 minutes

servings: 4 to 6

Ingredients

8 ounces penne, rotini, or other small pasta

1½ cups cooked or 1 (15.5-ouncecan chickpeas, drained and rinsed ½ cup pitted kalamata olives

½ cup minced oil-packed sun-dried tomatoes

1   (6-ouncejar marinated artichoke hearts, drained 2 jarred roasted red peppers, chopped

½ cup frozen peas, thawed 1 tablespoon capers

2   teaspoons dried chives ½ cup olive oil

¼ cup white wine vinegar ½ teaspoon dried basil

1 garlic clove, minced

Salt and freshly ground black pepper

Directions

1.   In a pot of boiling salted water, cook the pasta, stirring occasionally, until al dente, about 10 minutes. Drain well and transfer to a large bowl. Add the chickpeas, olives, tomatoes, artichoke hearts, roasted peppers, peas, capers, and chives. Toss gently and set aside.

2.   In a small bowl, combine the oil, vinegar, basil, garlic, sugar, and salt and black pepper to taste. Pour the dressing onto

the pasta salad and toss to combine. Serve chilled or at room temperature.

Tabbouleh Salad

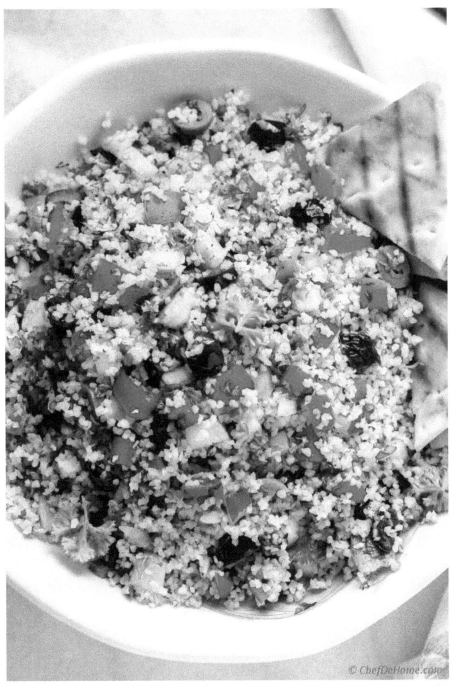

Preparation time: 15 minutes cooking time: 10 minutes servings: 4

Ingredients

1 cup whole-wheat couscous 1 cup boiling water

Zest and juice of 1 lemon 1 garlic clove, pressed Pinch sea salt

1 tablespoon olive oil, or flaxseed oil (optional

½ cucumber, diced small 1 tomato, diced small

1 cup fresh parsley, chopped

¼ cup fresh mint, finely chopped 2 scallions, finely chopped

4 tablespoons sunflower seeds (optional

Directions

1.   Put the couscous in a medium bowl, and cover with boiling water until all the grains are submerged. Cover the bowl with a plate or wrap. Set aside.

2.   Put the lemon zest and juice in a large salad bowl, then stir in the garlic, salt, and the olive oil (if using).

3.   Put the cucumber, tomato, parsley, mint, and scallions in the bowl, and toss them to coat with the dressing. Take the plate off the couscous and fluff with a fork.

4.   Add the cooked couscous to the vegetables, and toss to combine.

5.   Serve topped with the sunflower seeds (if using).

Nutrition Calories: 304; Total fat: 11g; Carbs: 44g; Fiber: 6g; Protein: 10g

Tuscan White Bean Salad

Preparation time: 10 minutes • marinating time: 30 minutes • servings: 2

Ingredients

For the dressing

1   tablespoon olive oil

2   tablespoons balsamic vinegar

1 teaspoon minced fresh chives, or scallions 1 garlic clove, pressed or minced

1 tablespoon fresh rosemary, chopped, or 1 teaspoon dried 1 tablespoon fresh oregano, chopped, or 1 teaspoon dried Pinch sea salt

For the salad

1 (14-ouncecan cannellini beans, drained and rinsed, or 1½ cups cooked 6 mushrooms, thinly sliced

1   zucchini, diced

2   carrots, diced

2 tablespoons fresh basil, chopped

Directions

1.   Make the dressing by whisking all the dressing ingredients together in a large bowl.

2.   Toss all the salad ingredients with the dressing. For the best flavor, put the salad in a sealed container, shake it vigorously, and leave to marinate 15 to 30 minutes.

Nutrition Calories: 360; Total fat: 8g; Carbs: 68g; Fiber: 15g; Protein: 18g

Indonesian Green BeanSalad With Cabbage And Carrots

Preparation time: 15 minutes cooking time: 0 minutes servings: 4

Ingredients

2 cups green beans, trimmed and cut into 1-inch pieces 2 medium carrots, cut into 1/4-inch slices

2 cups finely shredded cabbage

1/3 cup golden raisins

1/4 cup unsalted roasted peanuts

1 garlic clove, minced

1   medium shallot, chopped

1 1/2 teaspoons grated fresh ginger 1/3 cup creamy peanut butter

2   tablespoons soy sauce

2 tablespoons fresh lemon juice 1 teaspoon sugar(optional

1/4 teaspoon salt(optional 1/8 teaspoon ground cayenne

3/4 cup unsweetened coconut milk

Directions

1.   Lightly steam the green beans, carrots, and cabbage for about 5 minutes, then place them in a large bowl. Add the raisins and peanuts and set aside to cool.

2.   In a food processor or blender, puree the garlic, shallot, and ginger. Add the peanut butter, soy sauce, lemon juice, sugar,

salt, and cayenne, and process until blended. Add the coconut milk and blend until smooth. Pour the dressing over the salad, toss gently to combine, and serve.

4

Cucumber And Onion Quinoa Salad

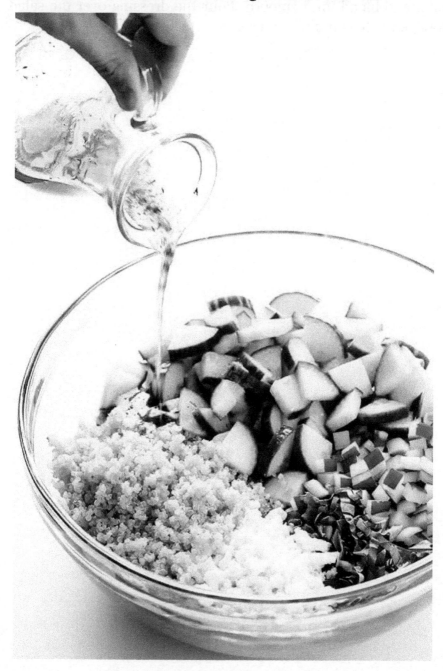

Preparation time: 15 minutes cooking time: 20 minutes servings: 4

Ingredients

1½ cups dry quinoa, rinsed and drained

2¼ cups water

⅓ cup white wine vinegar

2 tablespoons extra-virgin olive oil

1 tablespoon chopped fresh dill

1½ teaspoons vegan sugar

2 pinches salt

¼ teaspoon freshly ground black pepper

2 cups sliced sweet onions

2 cups diced cucumber 4 cups shredded lettuce

Directions

1.   In a medium pot, combine the quinoa and water. Bring to a boil.

2.   Cover, reduce the heat to medium-low, and simmer for 15 to 20 minutes, until the water is absorbed. Remove from the stove and let stand for 5 minutes. Fluff with a fork and set aside.

3.   Meanwhile, in a small bowl, mix the vinegar, olive oil, dill, sugar, salt, and pepper. Set aside. Into each of 4 wide-mouth jars, add 2 tablespoons of dressing, ½ cup of onions, ½ cup of cucumber, 1 cup of cooked quinoa, and 1 cup of shredded lettuce. Seal the lids tightly.

Nutrition: Calories: 369; Fat: 11g; Protein: 10g; Carbohydrates: 58g; Fiber: 6g; Sugar: 12g; Sodium: 88mg

Moroccan Aubergine Salad

Preparation time: 30 minutes cooking time: 15 minutes servings: 2

Ingredients

1 teaspoon olive oil

1 eggplant, diced

½ teaspoon ground cumin

½ teaspoon ground ginger

¼ teaspoon turmeric

¼ teaspoon ground nutmeg

Pinch sea salt

1 lemon, half zested and juiced, half cut into wedges 2 tablespoons capers

1   tablespoon chopped green olives 1 garlic clove, pressed

Handful fresh mint, finely chopped 2 cups spinach, chopped

Directions

1.

      Heat the oil in a large skillet on medium heat, then sauté the eggplant. Once it has softened slightly, about 5 minutes, stir in the cumin, ginger, turmeric, nutmeg, and salt. Cook until the eggplant is very soft, about 10 minutes.

2.   Add the lemon zest and juice, capers, olives, garlic, and mint. Sauté for another minute or two, to blend the flavors. Put a

handful of spinach on each plate, and spoon the eggplant mixture on top.

3.   Serve with a wedge of lemon, to squeeze the fresh juice over the greens.

4.   To tenderize the eggplant and reduce some of its naturally occurring bitter taste, you can sweat the eggplant by salting it. After dicing the eggplant, sprinkle it with salt and let it sit in a colander for about 30 minutes. Rinse the eggplant to remove the salt, then continue with the recipe as written.

Nutrition Calories: 97; Total fat: 4g; Carbs: 16g; Fiber: 8g; Protein: 4g

Potato Salad With Artichoke Hearts

Preparation time: 15 minutes cooking time: 15 minutes servings: 4 to 6

Ingredients

1½ pounds Yukon Gold potatoes, peeled and cut into 1-inch dice
1 (10-ouncepackage frozen artichoke hearts, cooked

2   cups halved ripe grape tomatoes ½ cup frozen peas, thawed

3   green onions, minced

1 tablespoon minced fresh parsley

⅓ cup olive oil

2   tablespoons fresh lemon juice 1 garlic clove, minced

Salt and freshly ground black pepper

Directions

1.   In a large pot of boiling salted water, cook the potatoes until just tender but still firm, about 15 minutes. Drain well and transfer to a large bowl.

2.   Quarter the artichokes and add them to the potatoes. Add the tomatoes, peas, green onions, and parsley and set aside.

3.   In a small bowl, combine the oil, lemon juice, garlic, and salt and pepper to taste. Mix well, pour the dressing over potato salad, and toss gently to combine. Set aside at room temperature to allow flavors to blend, about 20 minutes. Taste, adjusting seasonings if necessary, and serve.

Giardiniera

Preparation time: 15 minutes cooking time: 0 minutes servings: 6

Ingredients

1 medium carrot, cut into 1/4-inch rounds

1   medium red bell pepper, cut into 1/2-inch dice

1 cup small cauliflower florets

2   celery ribs, finely chopped

1/2 cup chopped onion

2 tablespoons salt (optional

1/4 cup sliced pimiento-stuffed green olives

1 garlic clove, minced

1/2 teaspoon sugar (optional

1/2 teaspoon crushed red pepper

1/4 teaspoon freshly ground black pepper

3 tablespoons white wine vinegar

1/3 cup olive oil

Directions

1.   In a large bowl, combine the carrot, bell pepper, cauliflower, celery, and onion. Stir in the salt and add enough cold water to cover. Tightly cover the bowl and refrigerate for 4 to 6 hours.

2.   Drain and rinse the vegetables and place them in a large bowl. Add the olives and set aside.

3.   In a small bowl, combine the garlic, sugar, crushed red pepper, black pepper, vinegar, and oil, and mix well. Pour the dressing over the vegetables and toss gently to combine. Cover and refrigerate overnight before serving.

Creamy Avocado-Dressed Kale Salad

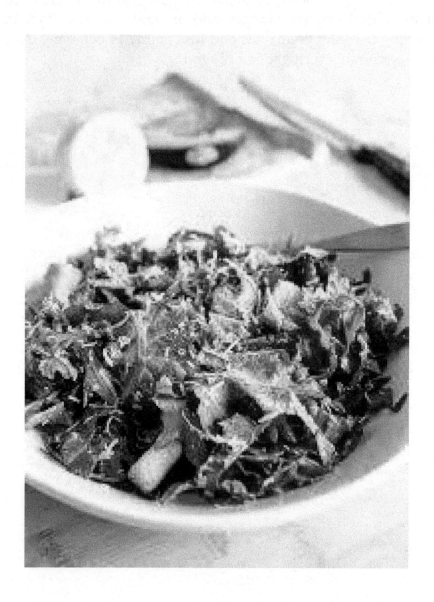

Preparation time: 10 minutes cooking time: 20 minutes servings: 4

Ingredients

For The Dressing

1 avocado, peeled and pitted

1 tablespoon fresh lemon juice, or 1 teaspoon lemon juice concentrate and 2 teaspoons water 1 tablespoon fresh or dried dill1 small garlic clove, pressed

1 scallion, chopped Pinch sea salt

¼ cup water

For The Salad

8 large kale leaves

½ cup chopped green beans, raw or lightly steamed 1 cup cherry tomatoes, halved

1   bell pepper, chopped 2 scallions, chopped

2   cups cooked millet, or other cooked whole grain, such as quinoa or brown rice Hummus (optional

Directions

To Make The Dressing

1.   Put all the ingredients in a blender or food processor. Purée until smooth, then add water as necessary to get the

consistency you're looking for in your dressing. Taste for seasoning, and add more salt if you need to.

To Make The Salad

2.   Chop the kale, removing the stems if you want your salad less bitter, and then massage the leaves with your fingers until it wilts and gets a bit moist, about 2 minutes. You can use a pinch salt if you like to help it soften. Toss the kale with the green beans, cherry tomatoes, bell pepper, scallions, millet, and the dressing. Pile the salad onto plates, and top them off with a spoonful of hummus (if using).

Nutrition Calories: 225; Total fat: 7g; Carbs: 37g; Fiber: 7g; Protein: 7g

Indonesian-Style Potato Salad

Preparation time: 10 minutes cooking time: 30 minutes servings: 4 to 6

Ingredients

Directions

1½ pounds small white potatoes, unpeeled 1 cup frozen peas, thawed

½ cup shredded carrot 4 green onions, chopped

1 tablespoon grapeseed oil 1 garlic clove, minced

⅓ cup creamy peanut butter ½ teaspoon Asian chili paste 2 tablespoons soy sauce

1 tablespoon rice vinegar

¾ cup unsweetened coconut milk

3 tablespoons chopped unsalted roasted peanuts, for garnish

1.   In a large pot of boiling salted water, cook the potatoes until tender, 20 to 30 minutes. Drain well and set aside to cool.

2.   When cool enough to handle, cut the potatoes into 1-inch chunks and transfer to a large bowl. Add the peas, carrot, and green onions, and set aside.

3.   In a small saucepan, heat the oil over medium heat. Add the garlic and cook until fragrant, about 30 seconds. Stir in the peanut butter, chili paste, soy sauce, vinegar, and about half of the coconut milk. Simmer over medium heat for 5 minutes, stirring frequently to make a smooth sauce. Add as much of the

remaining coconut milk as needed for a creamy consistency. Pour the dressing over the salad and toss well to combine. Garnish with peanuts and serve.

Roasted Beet and Avocado Salad

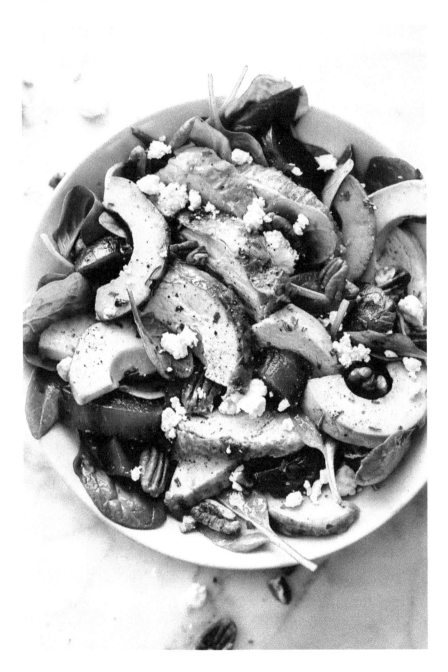

Preparation time: 10 minutes cooking time: 30minutes servings: 2

Ingredients

2 beets, peeled and thinly sliced

1 teaspoon olive oil

Pinch sea salt 1 avocado

2   cups mixed greens

3   to 4 tablespoons Creamy Balsamic Dressing

2 tablespoons chopped almonds, pumpkin seeds, or sunflower seeds (raw or toasted

Directions

1.   Preheat the oven to 400°F.

2.   Put the beets, oil, and salt in a large bowl, and toss the beets with your hands to coat. Lay them in a single layer in a large baking dish, and roast them in the oven 20 to 30 minutes, or until they're softened and slightly browned around the edges.

3.   While the beets are roasting, cut the avocado in half and take the pit out. Scoop the flesh out, as intact as possible, and slice it into crescents.

4.   Once the beets are cooked, lay slices out on two plates and top each beet slice with a similar-size avocado slice.

5.   Top with a handful of mixed greens. Drizzle the dressing over everything, and sprinkle on a few chopped almonds.

Nutrition Calories: 167; Total fat: 13g; Carbs: 15g; Fiber: 5g; Protein: 4g

Creamy Coleslaw

Preparation time: 10 minutes cooking time: 0 minutes servings: 4

Ingredients

1   small head green cabbage, finely shredded

1 large carrot, shredded

¾ cup vegan mayonnaise, homemade or store-bought

¼ cup soy milk

2   tablespoons cider vinegar ½ teaspoon dry mustard

¼ teaspoon celery seeds ½ teaspoon salt (optional

Freshly ground black pepper

Directions

1.   In a large bowl, combine the cabbage and carrot and set aside.

2.   In a small bowl, combine the mayonnaise, soy milk, vinegar, mustard, celery seeds, salt, and pepper to taste. Mix until smooth and well blended. Add the dressing to the slaw and mix well to combine. Taste, adjusting seasonings if necessary, and serve.

Sesame Cucumber Salad

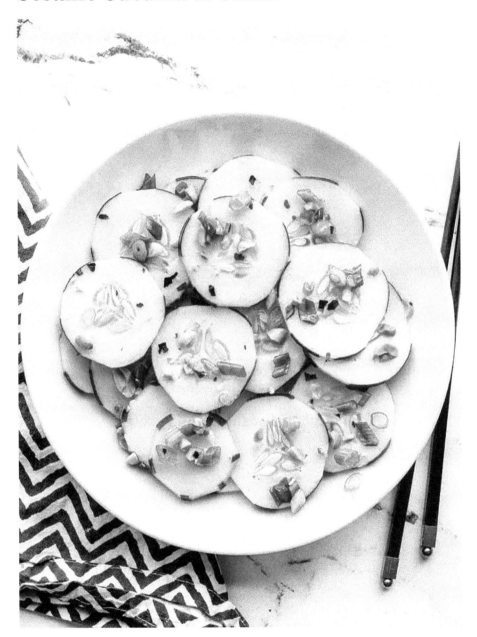

Preparation time: 15 minutes cooking time: 0 minutes

servings: 4 to 6

Ingredients

2   medium English cucumbers, peeled and cut into 1⁄4-inch slices 2 tablespoons chopped fresh parsley

3   tablespoons toasted sesame oil 2 tablespoons soy sauce

1   tablespoon mirin

2   teaspoons rice vinegar

1 teaspoon brown sugar (optional 2 tablespoons toasted sesame seeds

Directions

1.   In a small bowl, combine the cucumbers and parsley and set aside.

2.   In a separate small bowl, combine the oil, soy sauce, mirin, vinegar, and sugar, stirring to blend. Pour the dressing over the cucumbers. Set aside for at least 10 minutes.

3.   Spoon the cucumber salad into small bowls, sprinkle with sesame seeds, and serve.

Basil Mango Jicama Salad

Preparation Time: 15 Minutes • Chill Time: 60 Minutes • Servings:6

Ingredients

1   jicama, peeled and grated

1 mango, peeled and sliced

¼ cup non-dairy milk

2   tablespoons fresh basil, chopped

1 large scallion, chopped

⅛ teaspoon sea salt

1½ tablespoons tahini (optional)

Fresh greens (for serving)

Chopped cashews (optional, for serving)

Cheesy Sprinkle (optional, for serving)

Directions

1.   Put the jicama in a large bowl.

2.   Purée the mango in a food processor or blender, with just enough non-dairy milk to make a thick sauce.

3.   Add the basil, scallions, and salt. Stir in the tahini if you want to make a thicker, creamier, and more filling sauce.

4.   Pour the dressing over the jicama and marinate, covered in the fridge, for 1 hour or more to break down some of the starch.

Serve over a bed of greens, topped with chopped cashews and/or Cheesy Sprinkle (if using).

Per Serving Calories: 76; Total fat: 2g; Carbs: 14g; Fiber: 5g; Protein: 1g

Red Cabbage Slaw With Black-Vinegar Dressing

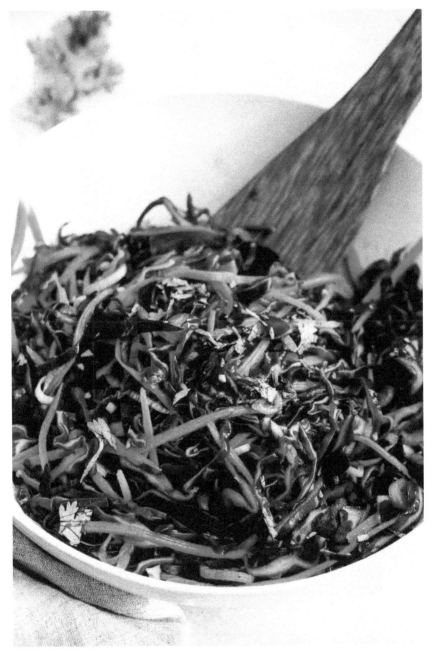

Preparation Time: 15 Minutes Cooking Time: 0 Minutes
Servings:6

Ingredients

4 cups shredded red cabbage

2 cups thinly sliced napa cabbage

1 cup shredded daikon radish

1/4 cup fresh orange juice

2 tablespoons Chinese black vinegar

1 tablespoon soy sauce

1 tablespoon grapeseed oil

 1 tablespoon toasted sesame oil

1 teaspoon grated fresh ginger

1/2 teaspoon ground Szechuan peppercorns

1 tablespoon black sesame seeds, for garnish

Directions

1.   In a large bowl, combine the red cabbage, napa, and daikon and set aside.

2.   In a small bowl, combine the orange juice, vinegar, soy sauce, grapeseed oil, sesame oil, ginger, and peppercorns. Blend well. Pour the dressing onto the slaw, stirring to coat. Taste, adjusting seasonings if necessary. Cover and refrigerate to allow flavors to blend, about 2 hours. Sprinkle with sesame seeds and serve.

Corn And Red Bean Salad

Preparation Time: 10 Minutes Cooking Time: 0 Minutes

Servings:4

Ingredients

1   (10-ounce) package frozen corn kernels, cooked

1½ cups cooked or 1 (15.5-ounce) can dark red kidney beans, drained and rinsed 1 celery rib, cut into ¼-inch slices

2   green onions, minced

2 tablespoons chopped fresh cilantro or parsley ¼ cup olive oil

2 tablespoons white wine vinegar ½ teaspoon ground cumin

¼ teaspoon sugar (optional) ½ teaspoon salt (optional)

⅛ teaspoon freshly ground black pepper

Directions

1.   In a large bowl, combine the corn, beans, celery, green onions, and cilantro, and set aside.

2.   In a small bowl, combine the oil, vinegar, cumin, sugar, salt, and pepper. Mix well and pour the dressing over the vegetables. Toss gently to combine and serve.

Greek Potato Salad

Preparation Time: 10 Minutes Cooking Time: 20 Minutes Servings:4

Ingredients

6 potatoes, scrubbed or peeled and chopped

Salt

¼ cup olive oil

2 tablespoons apple cider vinegar

2   tablespoons freshly squeezed lemon juice

1 teaspoon dried herbs

½ cucumber, chopped

¼ red onion, diced

¼ cup chopped pitted black olives

Freshly ground black pepper

Directions

1.   Put the potatoes in a large pot, add a pinch of salt, and pour in enough water to cover. Bring the water to

a boil over high heat. Cook the potatoes for 15 to 20 minutes, until soft. Drain and set aside to cool. (Alternatively, put the potatoes in a large microwave-safe dish with a bit of water. Cover and heat on high power for 10 minutes.)

2.   In a large bowl, whisk together the olive oil, vinegar, lemon juice, and dried herbs. Toss the cucumber, red onion, and olives with the dressing. Add the cooked, cooled potatoes, and toss to combine. Taste and season with salt and pepper as needed. Store leftovers in an airtight container in the refrigerator for up to 1 week.

Per Serving Calories: 358; Protein: 5g; Total fat: 16g; Saturated fat: 2g; Carbohydrates: 52g; Fiber: 5g

Rainbow Quinoa Salad

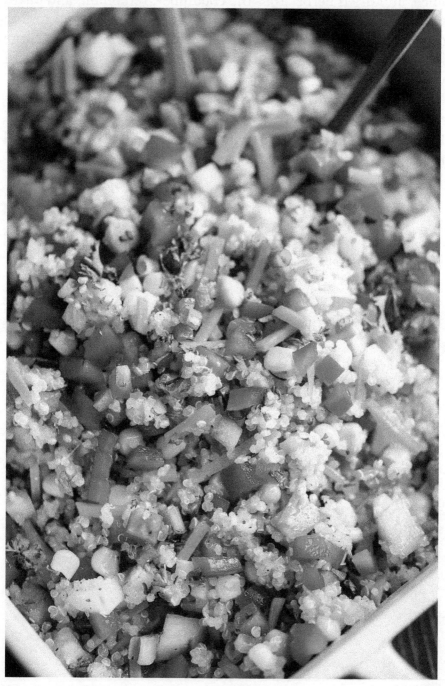

Preparation Time: 51 Minutes Cooking Time: 0 Minutes
Servings:6-8

Ingredients

3   tablespoons olive oil

Juice of 1½ lemons

1 teaspoon garlic powder

½ teaspoon dried oregano

1 bunch curly kale, stemmed and roughly chopped

2 cups cooked tricolor quinoa

1 cup canned mandarin oranges in juice, drained

1 cup diced yellow summer squash

1 red bell pepper, seeded and diced

½ red onion, thinly sliced

½ cup dried cranberries or cherries

½ cup slivered almonds

Directions

1.   In a small bowl, whisk together the oil, lemon juice, garlic
powder, and oregano.

2.   In a large bowl, toss the kale with the oil-lemon mixture
until well coated. Add the quinoa, oranges, squash, bell pepper,
and red onion and toss until all the ingredients are well combined.
Divide among bowls or transfer to a large serving platter. Top
with the cranberries and almonds.

Yellow Mung Bean Salad With Broccoli And Mango

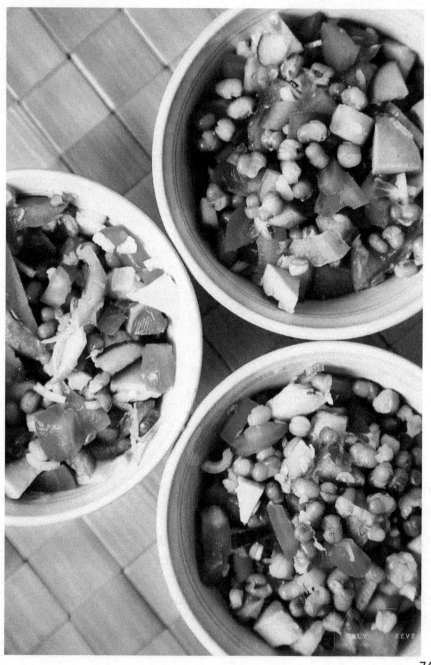

Preparation Time: 5 Minutes Cooking Time: 20 Minutes Servings:4

Ingredients

½ cup yellow mung beans, picked over, rinsed, and drained

3 cups small broccoli florets, blanched

1 ripe mango, peeled, pitted, and chopped

1 small red bell pepper, chopped

1 jalapeño or other hot green chile, seeded and minced

2 tablespoons chopped fresh cilantro

1 teaspoon grated fresh ginger

2 tablespoons fresh lemon juice

3 tablespoons grapeseed oil

⅓ cup unsalted roasted cashews, for garnish

Directions

1.   In a saucepan of boiling salted water, cook the mung beans until just tender, 18 to 20 minutes. Drain and run under cold water to cool. Transfer the beans to a large bowl. Add the broccoli, mango, bell pepper, chile, and cilantro. Set aside.

2.   In a small bowl, combine the ginger, lemon juice, oil. Stir to mix well, then pour the dressing over the vegetables and toss to combine. Sprinkle with cashews and serve.

Asian Slaw

Preparation Time: 15 Minutes Cooking Time: 0 Minutes
Servings:4

Ingredients

8 ounces napa cabbage, cut crosswise into ¼-inch strips

1 cup grated carrot

1   cup grated daikon radish

2 green onions, minced

2   tablespoons chopped fresh parsley

2 tablespoons rice vinegar

1   tablespoon grapeseed oil

2   teaspoons toasted sesame oil 1 tablespoon soy sauce

1   teaspoon grated fresh ginger ½ teaspoon dry mustard

Salt and freshly ground black pepper

2   tablespoons chopped unsalted roasted peanuts, for
garnish (optional)

Directions

1.   In a large bowl, combine the napa cabbage, carrot, daikon,
green onions, and parsley. Set aside.

2.   In a small bowl, combine the vinegar, grapeseed oil,
sesame oil, soy sauce, ginger, mustard, and salt and pepper to
taste. Stir until well blended. Pour the dressing over the
vegetables and toss gently to coat. Taste, adjusting seasonings if

necessary. Cover and refrigerate to allow flavors to blend, about 2 hours. Sprinkle with peanuts, if using, and serve.

The Great Green Salad

Preparation Time: 10 Minutes Cooking Time: 0 Minutes
Servings:

Ingredients

1 head Boston or Bibb lettuce

8 asparagus spears, trimmed and cut into 2-inch pieces

2 mini seedless cucumbers, sliced

1   small zucchini, cut into ribbons with potato peeler

1 avocado, peeled, pitted, and sliced

½ cup Green Goddess Dressing or store-bought vegan green
goddess dressing 2 scallions, thinly sliced

Directions

1.   Divide the lettuce leaves among 4 plates. Top each with
some of the asparagus, cucumber, zucchini, and avocado. Drizzle
each bowl with 2 tablespoons of dressing and sprinkle with
scallions.

Summer Berries With Fresh Mint

Preparation Time: 15 Minutes Cooking Time: 0 Minutes Servings:4 To 6

Ingredients

2   tablespoons fresh orange or pineapple juice

1 tablespoon fresh lime juice

1   tablespoon agave nectar

2   teaspoons minced fresh mint

2 cups pitted fresh cherries

1 cup fresh blueberries

1 cup fresh strawberries, hulled and halved

1/2 cup fresh blackberries or raspberries

Directions

1.   In a small bowl, combine the orange juice, lime juice, agave nectar, and mint. Set aside.

2.   In a large bowl, combine the cherries, blueberries, strawberries, and blackberries. Add the dressing and toss gently to combine. Serve immediately.

Curried Fruit Salad

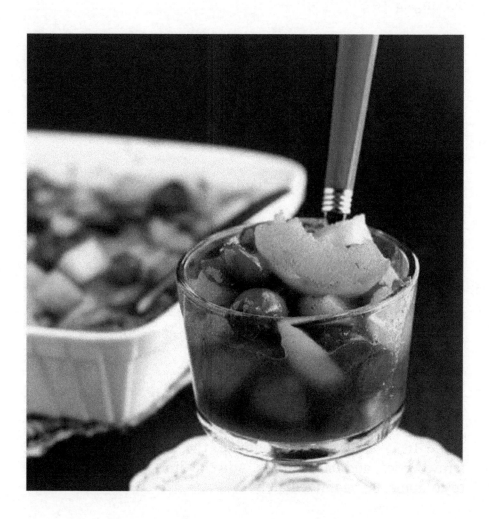

Preparation Time: 15 Minutes Cooking Time: 0 Minutes Servings:4 To 6

Ingredients

¾ cup vegan vanilla yogurt

¼ cup finely chopped mango chutney

1 tablespoon fresh lime juice

1 teaspoon mild curry powder

1   Fuji or Gala apple, cored and cut into ½-inch dice

2   ripe peaches, halved, pitted, and cut into ½-inch dice 4 ripe black plums, halved and cut into ¼-inch slices

1 ripe mango, peeled, pitted, and cut into ½-inch dice 1 cup red seedless grapes, halved

¼ cup unsweetened toasted shredded coconut ¼ cup toasted slivered almonds

Directions

1.   In a small bowl, combine the yogurt, chutney, lime juice, and curry powder and stir until well blended. Set aside.

2.   In a large bowl, combine the apple, peaches, plums, mango, grapes, coconut, and almonds. Add the dressing, toss gently to coat, and serve.

Stuffed Avocado

Preparation Time: 10 Minutes Cooking Time: 0 Minutes Servings:4

Ingredients

2 avocados, halved and pitted

1 (15-ounce) can black beans, rinsed and drained

1 cup frozen (and thawed) or fresh corn kernels

½ cup seeded and diced tomato

Juice of ½ lime

1   tablespoon maple syrup

1 teaspoon olive oil

2   pinches sea salt

2 pinches black pepper

1 tablespoon chopped fresh cilantro

Directions

1.   Scoop some avocado flesh from each half with a spoon, leaving a ¼- to ½-inch wall of avocado in the shell.

2.   In a large bowl, mix together the scooped-out avocado, beans, corn, tomato, lime juice, maple syrup, oil, salt, pepper, and cilantro until well incorporated.

3.   Spoon the filling into the avocado shells and enjoy.

Cranberry-Carrot Salad

Preparation Time: 15 Minutes Cooking Time: 0 Minutes
Servings:4

Ingredients

1 pound carrots, shredded

1   cup sweetened dried cranberries

1⁄2 cup toasted walnut pieces

2   tablespoons fresh lemon juice

3 tablespoons toasted walnut oil

1⁄8 teaspoon freshly ground black pepper

Directions

1.   In a large bowl, combine the carrots, cranberries, and walnuts. Set aside.

2.   In a small bowl, whisk together the lemon juice, walnut oil and pepper. Pour the dressing over the salad, toss gently to combine and serve.

Almond Crunch Chopped Kale Salad

Preparation Time: 10 Minutes Cooking Time: 10 Minutes
Servings:4

Ingredients

For The Dressing

¼ cup tahini

2 tablespoons Dijon mustard

2 tablespoons maple syrup

1   tablespoon lemon juice

¼ teaspoon salt

For The Almond Crunch

½ cup finely chopped raw almonds

2   teaspoons soy sauce or gluten-free tamari

1 teaspoon maple syrup

¼ teaspoon sea salt

For The Salad

1 bunch lacinato kale, stemmed and roughly chopped 1 green
apple, cored and thinly sliced

Directions

1.   Preheat the oven to 325°F. Line a baking sheet with parchment paper.

2.   To make the dressing: Whisk together all the dressing ingredients in a small bowl and set aside.

3.   To make the almond crunch: Mix together all the almond crunch ingredients in a medium bowl and

spread out evenly on the prepared baking sheet. Bake for 5 to 7 minutes, until slightly darker in color and crunchy. Let cool for 3 minutes.

4.   To make the salad: In a large bowl, mix together the kale and apples. Toss with the dressing and top with the almond crunch.

Apple-Sunflower Spinach Salad

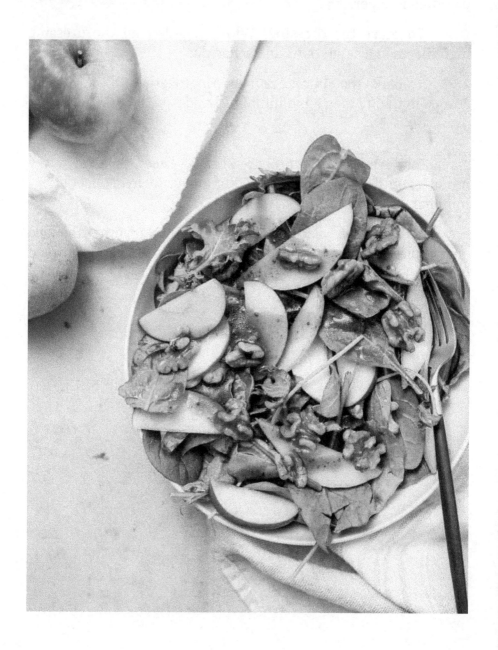

Preparation Time: 5 Minutes Cooking Time: 0 Minutes Servings:1

Ingredients

1   cup baby spinach

½ apple, cored and chopped

¼ red onion, thinly sliced (optional)

2   tablespoons   sunflower   seeds   or   Cinnamon-Lime
Sunflower Seeds 2 tablespoons dried cranberries

2 tablespoons Raspberry Vinaigrette

Directions

1.   Arrange the spinach on a plate. Top with the apple, red
onion (if using), sunflower seeds, and cranberries, and drizzle
with the vinaigrette.

Per Serving Calories: 444; Protein: 7g; Total fat: 28g; Saturated
fat: 3g; Carbohydrates: 53g; Fiber: 8g

Ruby Grapefruit and Radicchio Salad

Preparation Time: 10 Minutes Cooking Time: 0 Minutes Servings:4

Ingredients For The Salad

1 large ruby grapefruit

1 small head radicchio, torn into bite-size pieces

2 cups green leaf lettuce, torn into bite-size pieces

2 cups baby spinach

1 bunch watercress

4 to 6 radishes, sliced paper-thin

For The Dressing

juice of 1 lemon

2 teaspoons agave

1 teaspoon white wine vinegar

½ teaspoon sea salt

½ teaspoon freshly ground black pepper

¼ cup extra-virgin olive oil

Directions

1. To make the salad: Cut both ends off of the grapefruit, stand it on a cutting board on one of the flat sides, and, using a sharp knife, cut away the peel and all of the white pith. Remove the individual segments by slicing between the membrane and fruit on each side of each segment, dropping the fruit into a large salad bowl as you go. Add the radicchio, lettuce, spinach, watercress, and radishes to the bowl and toss well.

2. To make the dressing: Whisk together the lemon juice, agave, vinegar, salt, and pepper. Slowly whisk in the olive oil until the mixture is well combined and emulsified. Toss the salad with the dressing and serve immediately.

Darn Good Caesar Salad

Preparation Time: 10 Minutes Cooking Time: 0 Minutes Servings:4

Ingredients

For The Dressing

½ cup walnuts

½ cup water

3 tablespoons olive oil

Juice of ½ lime

1 tablespoon white miso paste

1 teaspoon soy sauce or gluten-free tamari

1 teaspoon Dijon mustard

1   teaspoon garlic powder

¼ teaspoon sea salt

½ teaspoon black pepper

For The Salad

2   heads romaine lettuce, chopped 1 cup cherry tomatoes, halved

Walnut Parmesan or store-bought vegan Parmesan, for garnish Vegan croutons, for garnish (optional)

Directions

1.　　To make the dressing: In a blender, combine all the dressing ingredients and blend until almost smooth, about 2 minutes. It's okay if this dressing is slightly chunky, which is more like a classic Caesar dressing texture.

2.　　To make the salad: In a large bowl, toss the lettuce with half of the dressing. Add more as desired. Divide among serving plates and top with the tomatoes and Parmesan. Finish the salad off with croutons, if desired.

Potato Salad Redux

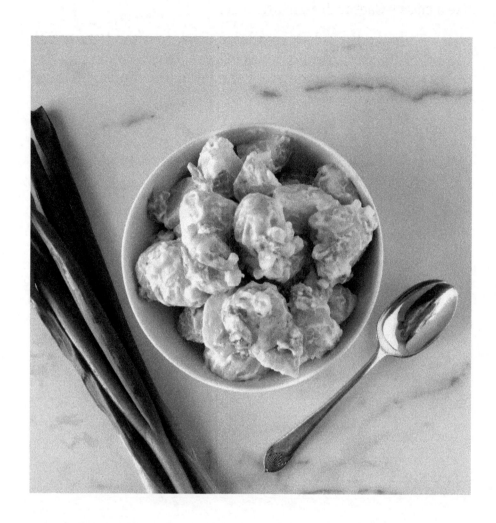

Preparation Time: 5 Minutes Cooking Time: 30 Minutes Servings:4 To 6

Ingredients

1½ pounds small white potatoes, unpeeled

2 celery ribs, cut into ¼-inch slices

¼ cup sweet pickle relish

3   tablespoons minced green onions

½ to ¾ cup vegan mayonnaise, homemade or store-bought

1 tablespoon soy milk

1   tablespoon tarragon vinegar 1 teaspoon

Dijon mustard

½ teaspoon salt (optional) Freshly ground black pepper

Directions

1.   In a large pot of salted boiling water, cook the potatoes until just tender, about 30 minutes. Drain and set aside to cool. When cool enough to handle, peel the potatoes and cut them into 1-inch dice. Transfer the

potatoes to a large bowl and add the celery, pickle relish, and green onions. Set aside.

2.   In a small bowl, combine the mayonnaise, soy milk, vinegar, mustard, salt, and pepper to taste. Mix until well blended. Pour the dressing onto the potato mixture, toss gently to combine, and serve.

Apple and Ginger Slaw

Preparation Time: 10 Minutes Cooking Time: 0 Minutes Servings:4

Ingredients

2   tablespoons olive oil

juice of 1 lemon, or 2 tablespoons prepared lemon juice

1 teaspoon grated fresh ginger

pinch of sea salt

2 apples, peeled and julienned

4 cups shredded red cabbage

Directions

1.   In a small bowl, whisk together the olive oil, lemon juice, ginger, and salt and set aside.

2.   In a large bowl, combine the apples and cabbage.

3.   Toss with the vinaigrette and serve immediately. Store leftovers in an airtight container in the refrigerator for up to 3 days.

Sunshine Fiesta Salad

Preparation Time: 15 Minutes Cooking Time: 0 Minutes Servings:4

Ingredients

For The Vinaigrette

Juice of 2 limes

1 tablespoon olive oil

1   tablespoon maple syrup or agave

¼ teaspoon sea salt

For The Salad

2   cups cooked quinoa

1 tablespoon Taco Seasoning or store-bought taco seasoning 2 heads romaine lettuce, roughly chopped

1 (15-ounce) can black beans, rinsed and drained 1 cup cherry tomatoes, halved

1 cup frozen (and thawed) or fresh corn kernels 1 avocado, peeled, pitted, and diced

4 scallions, thinly sliced 12 tortilla chips, crushed

Directions

1.   To make the vinaigrette: In a small bowl, whisk together all the vinaigrette ingredients.

2.   To make the salad: In a medium bowl, mix together the quinoa and taco seasoning. In a large bowl, toss the romaine with the vinaigrette. Divide among 4 bowls. Top each bowl with equal amounts quinoa, beans, tomatoes, corn, avocado, scallions, and crushed tortillas chips.

French-Style Potato Salad

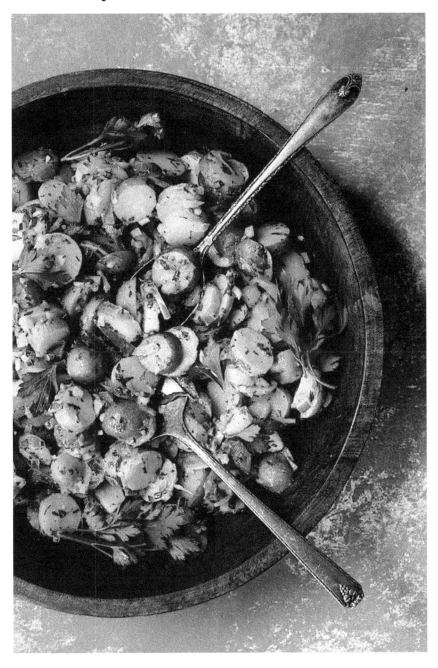

Preparation Time: 5 Minutes

Cooking Time: 30 Minutes Servings:4 To 6 Ingredients

Directions

1½ pounds small white potatoes, unpeeled

2 tablespoons minced fresh parsley

1 tablespoon minced fresh chives

1   teaspoon minced fresh tarragon or ½ teaspoon dried

⅓ cup olive oil

2   tablespoons white wine or tarragon vinegar ⅛ teaspoon freshly ground black pepper

1.   In a large pot of boiling salted water, cook the potatoes until tender but still firm, about 30 minutes. Drain and cut into ¼-inch slices. Transfer to a large bowl and add the parsley, chives, and tarragon. Set aside.

2.   In a small bowl, combine the oil, vinegar, pepper. Pour the dressing onto the potato mixture and toss gently to combine.

3.   Taste, adjusting seasonings if necessary. Chill for 1 to 2 hours before serving.

Roasted Carrot Salad

Preparation Time: 10 Minutes Cooking Time: 30 Minutes Servings:3

Ingredients

4 carrots, peeled and sliced

1 to 2 teaspoons olive oil or coconut oil

½ teaspoon ground cinnamon or pumpkin pie spice Salt

1 (15-ounce) can cannellini beans or navy beans, drained and rinsed

3 cups chopped hearty greens, such as spinach, kale, chard, or collards

⅓ cup dried cranberries or pomegranate seeds

⅓ cup slivered almonds or Cinnamon-Lime Sunflower Seeds

¼ cup Raspberry Vinaigrette or Cilantro-Lime Dressing, or 2 tablespoons freshly squeezed orange or lemon juice whisked with 2 tablespoons olive oil and a pinch of salt

Directions

1.

　　　　Preheat the oven or toaster oven to 400°F.

2.　　　In a medium bowl, toss the carrots with the olive oil and cinnamon and season to taste with salt. Transfer to a small tray, and roast for 15 minutes or until browned around the edges. Toss the carrots, add the beans, and roast for 15 minutes more. Let cool while you prep the salad. Divide the greens among three plates or containers, top with the cranberries and almonds, and add the roasted carrots and beans.

3.   Drizzle with the dressing of your choice. Store leftovers in an airtight container in the refrigerator for up to 1 week.

Roasted Potato Salad With Chickpeas And Tomatoes

Preparation Time: 5 Minutes Cooking Time: 20 Minutes Servings:4 To 6

Ingredients

1½ pounds Yukon Gold potatoes, cut into ½-inch dice

1 medium shallot, halved lengthwise and cut into ¼-inch slices ¼ cup olive oil

Salt and freshly ground black pepper 3 tablespoons white wine vinegar

1½ cups cooked or 1 (15.5-ounce) can chickpeas, drained and rinsed ⅓ cup chopped drained oil-packed sun-dried tomatoes

¼ cup green olives, pitted and halved ¼ cup chopped fresh parsley

Directions

1.   Preheat the oven to 425°F. In a large bowl, combine the potatoes, shallot, and 1 tablespoon of the oil. Season with salt and pepper to taste and toss to coat. Transfer the potatoes and shallot to a baking sheet and roast, turning once, until tender and golden brown, about 20 minutes. Transfer to a large bowl and set aside to cool.

2.   In a small bowl, combine the remaining 3 tablespoons oil with the vinegar and pepper to taste. Add the chickpeas, tomatoes, olives, and parsley to the cooked potatoes and shallots. Drizzle with the dressing and toss gently to combine. Taste, adjusting seasonings if necessary. Serve warm or at room temperature.

Spinach and Pomegranate Salad

Preparation Time: 10 Minutes Cooking Time: 0 Minutes
Servings:4

Ingredients

10 ounces baby spinach seeds from 1 pomegranate

1 cup fresh blackberries

¼ red onion, thinly sliced

½ cup chopped pecans

¼ cup balsamic vinegar

¾ cup olive oil

½ teaspoon sea salt

½ teaspoon freshly ground black pepper

Directions

1.   In a large bowl, combine the spinach, pomegranate seeds, blackberries, red onion, and pecans.

2.   In a small bowl, whisk together the vinegar, olive oil, salt, and pepper. Toss with the salad and serve immediately.

Cobb Salad with Portobello Bacon

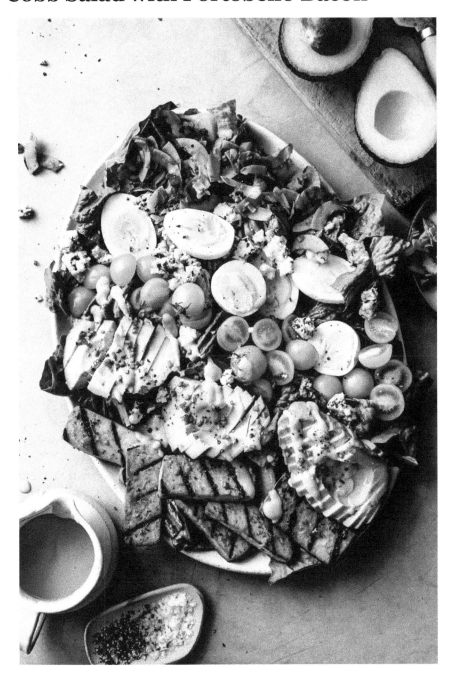

Preparation Time: 15 Minutes Cooking Time: 0 Minutes Servings:4

Ingredients

2 heads romaine lettuce, finely chopped

1 pint cherry tomatoes, halved

1 avocado, peeled, pitted, and diced

1 cup frozen (and thawed) or fresh corn kernels

1 large cucumber, peeled and diced

Portobello Bacon or store-bought vegan bacon

4 scallions, thinly sliced

Unhidden Valley Ranch

Dressing or store-bought vegan ranch dressing

Directions

1.   Scatter a layer of romaine in the bottom of each of 4 salad bowls. With the following ingredients, create lines that cross the top of the romaine, in this order: tomatoes, avocado, corn, cucumber, and portobello bacon.

2.   Sprinkle with the scallions and drizzle with ranch dressing.

German-Style Potato Salad

Preparation Time: 15 Minutes Cooking Time: 0 Minutes
Servings:4 To 6

Ingredients

1½ pounds white potatoes, unpeeled

½ cup olive oil

4 slices tempeh bacon, homemade or store-bought

1 medium bunch green onions, chopped

1 tablespoon whole-wheat flour

2 tablespoons sugar

⅓ cup white wine vinegar

¼ cup water

½ teaspoon salt

⅛ teaspoon freshly ground black pepper

Directions

1.   In a large pot of boiling salted water, cook the potatoes until just tender, about 30 minutes. Drain well and set aside to cool.

2.   In a large skillet, heat the oil over medium heat. Add the tempeh bacon and cook until browned on both sides, about 5 minutes total. Remove from skillet, and set aside to cool.

3.   Cut the cooled potatoes into 1-inch chunks and place in a large bowl. Crumble or chop the cooked tempeh bacon and add to the potatoes.

4.   Reheat the skillet over medium heat. Add the green onions and cook for 1 minute to soften. Stir in the flour, sugar, vinegar, water, salt, and pepper, and bring to a boil, stirring until smooth. Pour the hot dressing onto the potatoes. Stir gently to combine and serve.

Sweet Pearl Couscous Salad with Pear & Cranberries

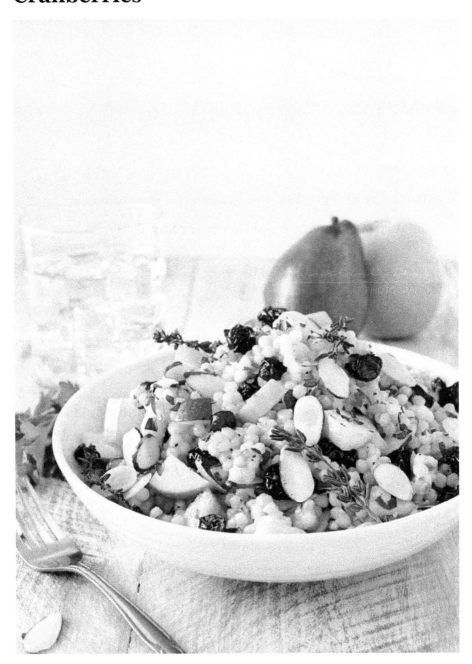

Preparation Time: 5 Minutes Cooking Time: 10 Minutes Servings:4

Ingredients

1 cup pearl couscous

1½ cups water

Salt

¼ cup olive oil

¼ cup freshly squeezed orange juice

1   tablespoon sugar, maple syrup, or Simple Syrup

1 pear, cored and diced

½ cucumber, diced

¼ cup dried cranberries or raisins

Directions

1.   In a small pot, combine the couscous, water, and a pinch of salt. Bring to a boil over high heat, turn the heat to low, and cover the pot. Simmer for about 10 minutes, until the couscous is al dente.

2.   Meanwhile, in a large bowl, whisk together the olive oil, orange juice, and sugar. Season to taste with salt and whisk again to combine.

3.   Add the pear, cucumber, cranberries, and cooked couscous. Toss to combine. Store leftovers in an airtight container in the refrigerator for up to 1 week.

Per Serving Calories: 365; Protein: 6g; Total fat: 14g; Saturated fat: 2g; Carbohydrates: 55g; Fiber: 4g